28 DAY FERTILITY DIET

PAVLA KESSLEROVA

DEDICATION

To Ebony and Tapiwa

CONTENTS

This book contains 4 chapters for the 4 different phases of the cycle (Menstruation, Follicular phase, Ovulation and Luteal Phase) with one recipe for each day of the week.

The aim is to eat food which will help to detoxify and cleanse the body and deliver the right nutrition and vitamins to help the system get ready for conception. **I can't stress more how important it is to eat strictly organic food.** As I mentioned in my previous book, there are studies confirming that pesticides which are used on almost every piece of non organic vegetable and fruit may actually cause endometriosis, a condition which may lead to infertility. Also hormones used in genetically modified food may interfere with your hormonal balance lowering your chances to conceive. Cooking with brown pasta, brown rice, organic flour, staying away from processed foods, alcohol and making sure you get enough whole grains and lean protein is essential.

Lots and lots of vitamin C. As explained in my book " 5 Simple Steps To Fertility" **Vitamin C deficiency is proved to be linked to infertility.** Just get enough vitamin C as this will help at all stages including preconception, pregnancy, child birth and even beyond.

Please remember to deliver only the best to your body during the time you are trying to conceive. The rules are simple. Read the ingredients on the packet. As soon an item contains too many (usually more then 5) ingredients and has E number this, E number that … you might want to avoid those foods. You don't need artificial colors, preservatives or coloring in your system. It is messing up with your natural hormonal balance.

Drink water and lots of it.

For breakfast choose organic fruit with cereals and your lunch should be all about salads. Blueberries, raspberries, grapes, almonds or other packs of mixed nuts are good snacks. You will see just after a week on fresh food how your mood will change and how much happier you will feel. The body reacts immediately when is treated nicely, it pays you back. It's a simple deal, if we are providing bad stuff we shouldn't expect the body to be strong and fit.

Try to eat like our great grandparents used to eat. Fresh from the butcher, fresh from the local farm, fresh from the market. No colorants, no chemicals, no preservatives. Did they have so much cancer? No. Did they have so many issues with fertility? No.

Aspartame is definitely to be avoided. All chewing gums and diet drinks are sugar free, because they are containing artificial sweeteners which our body is not equipped to deal with. Liver can't break it down unlike a natural sugars which we are designed to use as a natural fuel.

If you are prepared to try everything as I was, staying away from junk and processed food is the easiest first step.

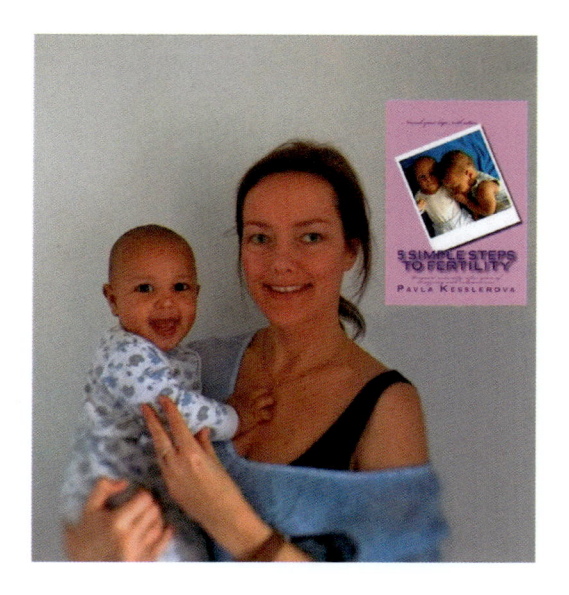

I like things simple, for that reason I write short straight to the point books, as the process is not complex. You have asked me what I was eating, so here is my 4 week diet. My diet was vegetarian so I adjusted some recipes for meat lovers. My breakfasts and snacks were always the same: grapes, cereals, blueberries, raspberries, watermelon, almonds, nuts and salads. Feel free to improvise and alternate your dishes to your liking, this is not a bible to be followed religiously, this is just a guide which will hopefully be a useful tool on your journey to pregnancy.

Good luck and Bon appetite!

1 *MENSTRUATION*

Menstruation is all about foods rich in iron: Meat, beans, fish, leafy green vegetables and seeds. Iron and protein are important if you have endometriosis or bleed heavily. Food with anti-inflammatory properties (fish, seeds and leafy greens) can help control cramps by encouraging healthy blood flow. Eat plenty other food sources that are high in vitamin C which helps the body absorb iron from food.

Avoid cold foods (if your periods are clotted and painful) and alcohol, caffeine and spicy foods, which can make bleeding even heavier.

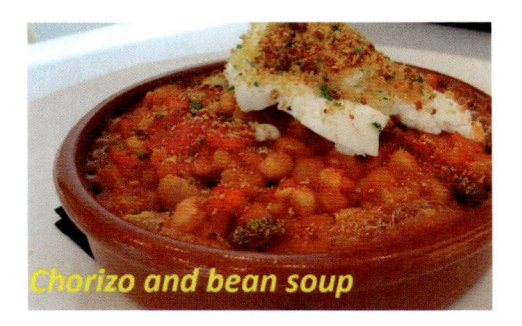

Chorizo and bean soup

Chorizo and bean soup

- 1 tablespoon organic olive oil or organic rapeseed oil
- 2 chorizo sausages (or bacon instead), sliced
- 1 red chilli, chopped
- 1 organic red pepper, diced
- 1 garlic clove, crushed

- 1 (300g) tin cannellini or other beans, drained and rinsed
- 1 (400g) organic fresh or tin chopped tomatoes
- 1 stock cube, diluted in about 240ml water
- 1 small bunch fresh parsley and basil, finely chopped (optional)
- 1 tablespoon grated Parmesan cheese (optional)

Method

1. Heat the oil in a pan, add the sausage, chilli, red pepper and garlic, keep on a medium heat for 5 minutes, stirring occasionally.

2. Add the beans, tomatoes, stock and bring to the boil, simmer for a further 5 to 10 minutes until reduced a little.
3. Serve in warmed bowls, top with fresh herbs and Parmesan if you like.

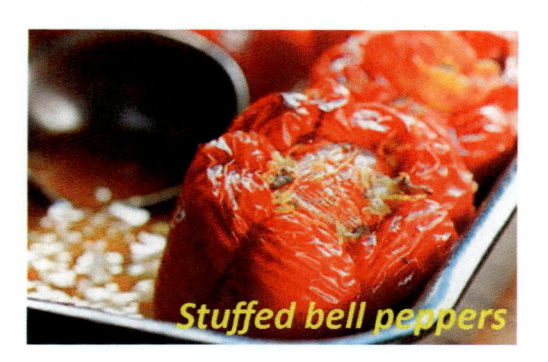

Stuffed bell peppers

Stuffed bell peppers

- 4 organic bell peppers, any color
- Salt
- 5 Tbsp organic extra-virgin olive oil
- 1 medium organic yellow onion, peeled and chopped
- 1 clove of garlic, peeled and chopped
- 500g of organic lean ground beef
- 1 1/2 cup of **cooked brown** rice
- 1 cup chopped tomatoes, organic fresh or canned (if using can, drain of excess liquid first)
- 1 teaspoon of oregano
- Fresh ground pepper
- 1/2 cup ketchup
- 1/2 tsp of Worcestershire Sauce
- Dash of Tabasco sauce

Method

1. Bring a large pot of water to a boil over high heat. Meanwhile, cut top off peppers 1 inch from the stem end and remove seeds. Add several generous pinches of salt to boiling water. Add peppers and boil, using a spoon to keep peppers completely submerged, until their flesh slightly softened, about 3 minutes. Drain, set aside to cool.
2. Preheat oven to 180°C. Heat 4 tbsp of the oil in a large frying pan over medium heat. Add onions and cook, stirring often, until soft and translucent, about 5 minutes. Add the garlic and cook a minute more. Remove from heat, add meat, rice, tomatoes, and oregano, and season generously with salt and pepper. Mix well. It is easier to put the ingredients at this point into a large bowl and mix together with your hands.
3. Drizzle remaining 1 tablespoon of olive oil inside the peppers. Arrange the cut side of the peppers up in a baking dish, then stuff peppers with filling. Combine ketchup, Worcestershire sauce, Tabasco sauce, and 1/4 cup of water in a small bowl, then spoon over filling. Add 1/4 cup of water to the baking dish. Place in oven and bake for 40-50 minutes (or longer, depending on how big the peppers are that you are stuffing), until the internal temperature of the stuffed peppers is 70-80°C

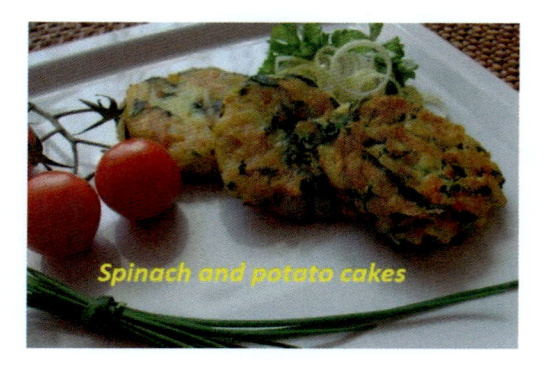

Spinach and potato cakes

Spinach and potato cakes

- 1 large organic potato, peeled and grated
- 150g self raising flour
- 2 free-range eggs
- 70ml milk
- Handful spinach, shredded
- pinch grated nutmeg
- salt and freshly ground black pepper
- 25g butter
- 1 tbsp organic olive oil
- 1 lemon, juice only

Method

1. Place the grated potato, flour, eggs, and milk into a bowl and mix until well combined. Add more milk as necessary until the mixture is of dropping consistency.
2. Add the spinach and nutmeg and stir until well combined. Season, to taste, with salt and freshly ground black pepper.
3. Heat the butter and oil in a frying pan over a medium heat. Add spoonfuls of the spinach mixture and fry for 3-4 minutes on each side, or until golden-brown on both sides and heated through. Remove from the pan

using a slotted spoon and set aside to drain on kitchen paper.
4. To serve, stack the spinach and potato cakes onto a serving plate and squeeze over the lemon juice.

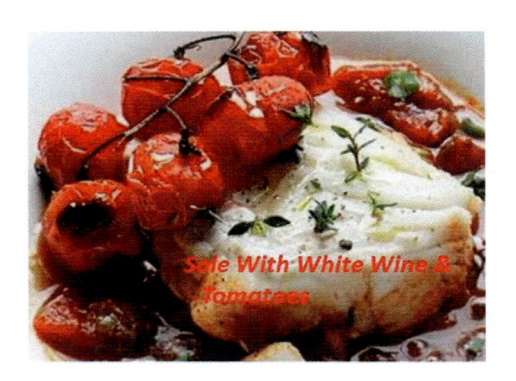

Sole With White Wine & Tomatoes

- 2 tablespoons organic extra virgin olive oil
- 1 tablespoon minced garlic
- 1/3 cup dry white wine
- 250g organic cherry tomatoes
- 400g mixed heirloom tomatoes, stemmed and coarsely chopped
- 1 tablespoon butter
- Salt and ground black pepper
- 400g sole filets
- 1/2 tablespoon thinly sliced basil, for garnish (optional)

Method

1. In a large skillet or sauté pan, warm the olive oil over medium heat. Add the garlic; cook, stirring, until it just begins to color, about 3 minutes. Add the white wine and cook for about 2 minutes.
2. Add the cherry tomatoes and cook, stirring often, until they just begin to burst and release some of their juices, about 5 minutes. Add the chopped tomatoes, and cook about 3 minutes more. Stir in the butter, and season with salt and pepper.
3. Sprinkle the sole with salt and pepper, and nestle the filets in the sauce. Cover the pan and cook until the fish is just opaque throughout, about 4-5 minutes.
4. Spoon the sauce over the fish and serve immediately with crusty bread, garnishing with fresh basil, if desired.

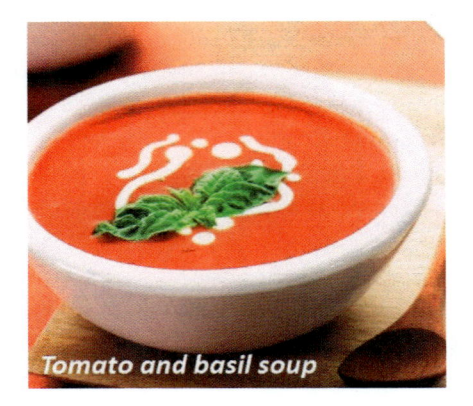

Tomato and basil soup

Tomato and basil soup

- 1 tin organic chopped tomatoes
- 200ml chicken or vegetable stock
- 1 tablespoon sugar
- 18 leaves fresh basil
- 2 tablespoons butter
- 125ml whipping or double cream
- 2 teaspoons salt

Method

1. Simmer the tomatoes and stock for 10 minutes.
2. Add sugar and basil and cook for a further 5 minutes. Add more sugar if required.
3. Stir in cream and butter until the butter has melted. Blend slightly and season to taste.

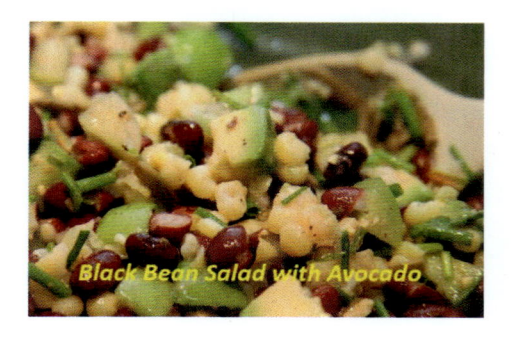

Black Bean Salad with Avocado

- 2 cans black beans, rinsed and drained
- 3 ears fresh cooked corn, kernels cut off the cob
- 2 organic red bell peppers, diced
- 2 cloves garlic, minced
- 2 tablespoons minced shallots
- 1 teaspoon sesame seeds
- 2 teaspoons salt
- 1/4 teaspoon cayenne pepper
- 2 tablespoons sugar
- 9 tablespoons extra virgin olive oil
- 1 teaspoon lime zest
- 6 tablespoons fresh lime juice
- 1/2 cup chopped fresh cilantro
- 2 avocados, chopped

Method

1. Combine all ingredients except for avocados in a large bowl and mix well. Cover and chill for a few hours or overnight. Right before serving, add avocados and mix gently, being careful not to mash. avocados. Garnish with a more chopped cilantro if desired. Serve at room temperature.

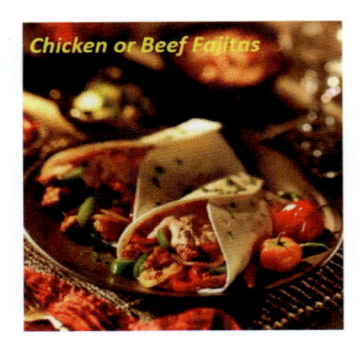

Chicken or Beef Fajitas

- 500 skirt steak or other beef or chicken easily cut into strips
- 1 small onion, sliced,
- 1 large Bell pepper, sliced
- 1/4 cup soy sauce
- 1/4 cup lime juice
- 1/2 teaspoon chili powder
- 2 Tablespoons oil
- salsa, sour cream and tortillas

Method

1. Combine soy sauce, lime juice, chili powder, and oil.
2. Slice the meat into small slices.
3. Marinate everything together in a bowl or plastic bag for at least 15min.
4. Add a little oil to the skillet and get it very hot (the oil will shimmer otherwise the meat will steam instead of browning). When the meat is browned, remove and add veggies. When they begin to soften, return meat to skillet to heat through.
5. Serve with salsa, sour cream and tortillas.

2 *FOLLICULAR PHASE*

During the follicular phase estrogen levels are on the rise as your body is working hard to develop a dominant follicle.

You should eat food containing a phytonutrient called di-indolylmethane (DIM), which can help metabolize estrogen better. In fact, DIM binds to environmental estrogens like pesticides and hormones in meat and dairy products, helping rid the body of excess estrogen. This week is time for broccoli, kale, cabbage, cauliflower, avocado, nuts, seeds and leafy greens. These foods are loaded with vitamin E, which is found in the fluid of the follicle that's housing your egg.

Avoid alcohol as it affects hormonal balance and is dehydrating. The loss of water in the body may make cervical mucus too thick.

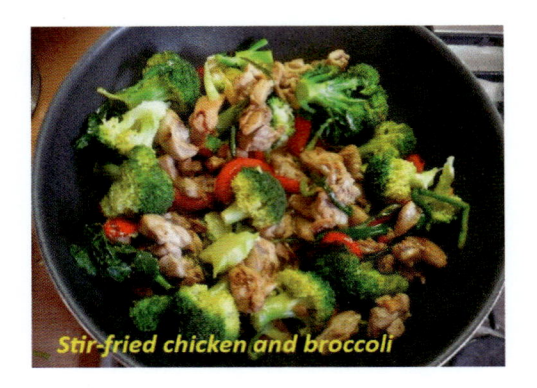

Stir-fried chicken and broccoli

- 500g organic chicken breast strips
- 2 tbsp. organic rapeseed oil
- 4 cup organic vegetables (broccoli, red & green peppers strips, sliced water chestnuts)
- 1 1/2 cup chicken broth
- 3 tbsp. soy sauce
- 3 tbsp. cornstarch
- 2 tsp. brown sugar
- 1 1/2 cup organic brown rice

Method

1. Stir fry chicken in hot oil in large skillet until brown. Add vegetables; stir until done. Mix broth, soy, cornstarch and sugar. Add to skillet. Boil, continue for 2 minutes. Prepare rice. Serve chicken mixture over hot rice.

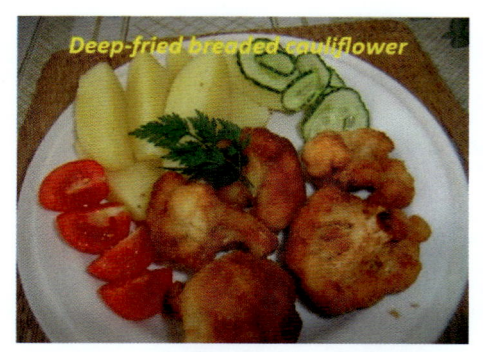

Deep-fried breaded cauliflower

- 1 small head of cauliflower cut into small pieces
- 1 cup flour
- ½ cup cornstarch
- 1 tsp baking powder
- ½ tsp salt
- 1 cup water
- 2 cups breadcrumbs
- Organic oil for frying
- Boiled potatoes

Method

1. In a large bowl mix flour, baking powder, cornstarch and salt. Add water, hot sauce and mix until the batter is smooth.
2. Dip cauliflower pieces into the batter and coat evenly. Allow excess batter to drip off. Roll the cauliflower in breadcrumbs until coated thoroughly.
3. Heat deep fryer to 365° F / 185° C. Deep fry cauliflower pieces in batches until golden brown. Drain on paper towels. Serve with potatoes and garnish.

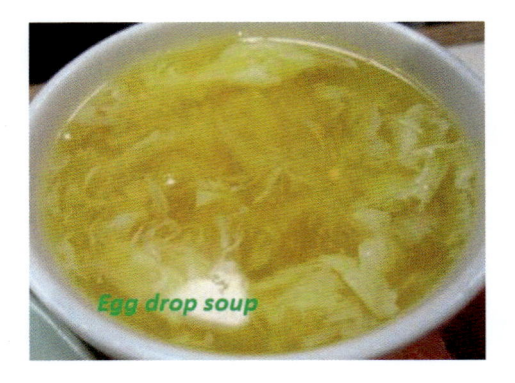

Egg drop soup

Egg drop soup

- 4 cups chicken broth or stock
- 2 organic eggs, lightly beaten
- 1 -2 green onions, minced
- 1/4 teaspoon white pepper
- Salt to taste
- A few drops of sesame oil (optional)

Method

1. In a wok or saucepan, bring the 4 cups of chicken broth to a boil. Add the white pepper and salt, and the sesame oil if using. Cook for about another minute.
2. Very slowly pour in the eggs in a steady stream. To make shreds, stir the egg rapidly in a clockwise direction for one minute. To make thin streams or ribbons, gently stir the eggs in a clockwise direction until they form.
3. Garnish with green onion and serve.

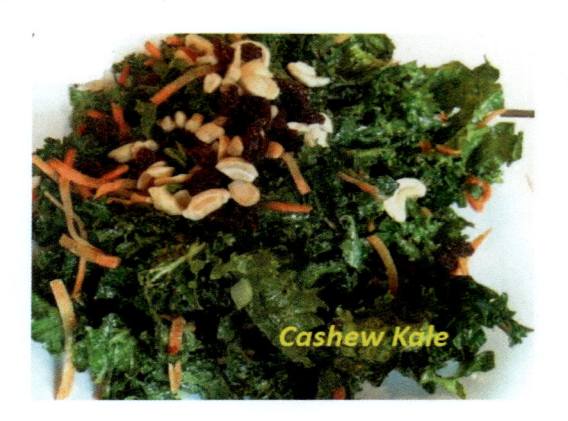

Cashew Kale

Cashew Kale

- 2 tablespoons olive oil
- 1 large carrot, thinly sliced into rounds (about 1/2 cup)
- 2 bunches kale, thick stems removed, thinly sliced (about 8 cups)
- 1 garlic clove, minced
- 2 to 3 tablespoons tamari (soy sauce)
- 1/2 cup raw cashews
- 1/4 cup raisins

Method

1. Heat the olive oil over medium heat and sauté the carrot for five minutes. Add the garlic, kale, tamari, cashews and raisins and sauté a few minutes until cashews begin to soften.5 minutes. Add the garlic and cook a minute more.

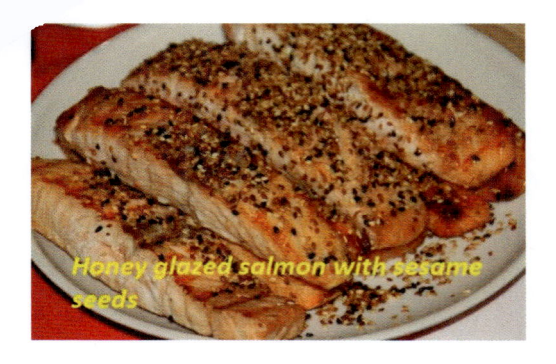

Honey glazed salmon with sesame seeds

Honey glazed salmon with sesame seeds

- 2 tbsp extra virgin olive oil
- 2 salmon fillets
- 4 tsp clear organic honey
- 1 tbsp balsamic vinegar
- 4 tsp sesame seeds
- Fresh vegetables and mashed potato

Method

1. Heat the oil in a frying pan and once it's nice and hot, add the salmon fillets and fry for 2-3 minutes each side.
2. With the salmon still in the pan, drain the oil and add the honey and balsamic vinegar. Cook for 2-3 more minutes.
3. Cover the salmon fillets with honey and sesame seeds and take the salmon out of the pan.
4. Serve with fresh vegetables and mashed potato.

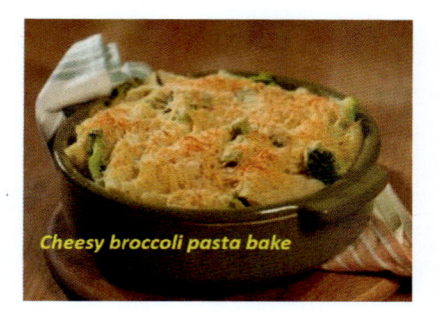
Cheesy broccoli pasta bake

Cheesy broccoli pasta bake

- 0,5l milk
- 1 garlic cloves, bashed
- 2 bay leaves
- 250g dried brown pasta
- 200g organic broccoli, in small florets
- 45g butter
- 45g plain flour
- a little freshly grated nutmeg
- 1/2 tsp mustard powder
- small bunch parsley, roughly chopped
- 150g cheese, grated (Cheddar, Parmesan, Gruyère, or a mixture)

Method

1. Bring the milk, garlic and bay leaves to the boil in a small saucepan, then remove from the heat and leave to infuse. Cook the pasta to al dente following pack instructions (if you're freezing, cook for 1 min less), adding the broccoli for the final 2 min. Drain.
2. Strain the milk into a jug. Heat the butter in the pan until foaming then stir in the flour for 1 min. Add the milk a little at a time, stirring or whisking constantly to remove any lumps. Bubble for 1-2 min, stirring

constantly until you have a thick, lump-free sauce.

3. Remove from the heat and stir in some nutmeg, the mustard powder, parsley, three-quarters of the cheese and seasoning. Combine with the pasta and broccoli and transfer to one large, or individual, heatproof dishes. Scatter over the remaining cheese and heat the grill to high and cook for 2-3 min until golden and bubbling.

3 *OVULATION*

Near ovulation plenty of B vitamins and other nutrients are required to support the release of the egg and promote implantation.

Zinc can help with cell division and progesterone production.

Vitamin C is found in high quantities in the follicle after the egg is released and may play a role in progesterone production as well.

Drink lots of water. Water plays a key role in transporting hormone and developing follicles. It also helps thin out cervical mucus, which may make it a little easier for the sperms to get to their goal.

Essential fatty acids (EFAs) are crucial during this phase, as they promoting blood flow to the uterus and supporting the opening of the follicle to release the egg.

Have some chocolate this week, it is well known aphrodisiac.

Avoid acidic foods like coffee, alcohol and processed foods, which may make your cervical mucus hostile to sperm.

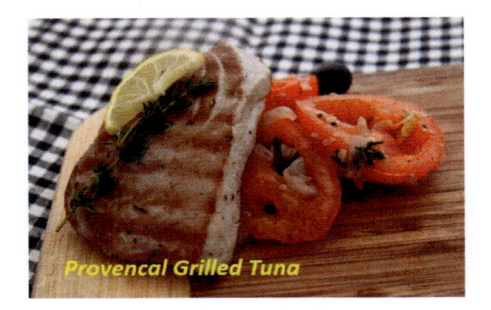

Provencal Grilled Tuna

Provencal Grilled Tuna

- 1-1/2 cups chopped seeded tomatoes
- 3/4 cup chopped fresh parsley
- 1/4 cup chopped pitted olives
- 1 Tablespoon white wine vinegar
- 1/4 teaspoon dried tarragon, crushed
- 1/4 teaspoon salt
- 2 cloves garlic, minced
- 4 smaller tuna steaks or two large
- 1-1/2 teaspoons dried Herbs de Provence
- 1/4 teaspoon salt
- Cooking spray
- 8 chive sprigs, loosely chopped

Method

1. Combine tomato, parsley, olives, vinegar, tarragon , salt, and garlic in a medium bowl. Cover and chill for 20 minutes.
2. Prepare your grill. Sprinkle tune with Herbs de Provence and 1/4 teaspoon salt. Cover grill rack with cooking spray. Place fish on sprayed grill rack. Cook 3 minutes on each side or until fish is medium rare or desired degree of doneness.

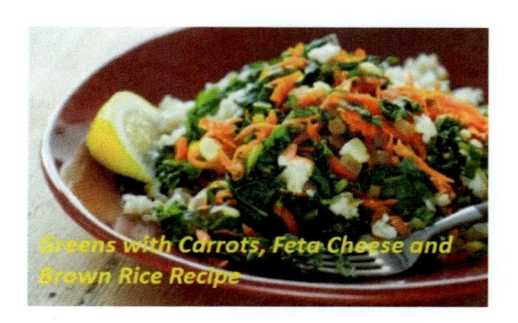

Greens with Carrots, Feta Cheese and Brown Rice Recipe

Greens with Carrots, Feta Cheese and Brown Rice Recipe

- 2 organic carrots, shredded
- 2 bunches dark leafy greens (kale, collard greens or Swiss chard), tough stems removed, leaves very thinly sliced
- 1/2 red onion, finely chopped
- 1/4 teaspoon sea salt
- 1/2 teaspoon ground black pepper
- 1/4 pound feta cheese, crumbled
- 1or 1,5 cup of organic Whole Grain Brown Rice, prepared according to package directions

Method

1. Put carrots, greens, onions, 1/4 cup water, salt and pepper into a large, deep skillet and toss well. Cover and cook over medium heat, tossing once or twice, until greens are wilted and tender, 10 to 15 minutes. Toss with feta cheese and spoon over brown rice.

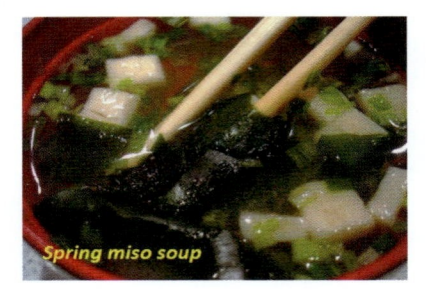

Spring miso soup

Spring miso soup

- 20g instant dashi (Japanese stock) or 3 tsp good quality vegetable bouillon powder
- 800ml boiling water
- 4 spring onions
- 2 tbsp white or red miso paste
- 1 tbsp sweet rice wine
- 1 tbsp soya sauce
- 200g silken tofu, cubed

Method

1. Put the dashi or bouillon powder with the boiling water in a saucepan, and stir well.
2. Finely slice the asparagus on the diagonal and add to the pan. Simmer for three minutes.
3. Place the miso paste in a small bowl and add a ladleful of the hot broth, whisking with a small whisk to get rid of any lumps. When smooth, slowly pour the mixture back into the saucepan, whisking constantly.
4. Add the wine, soy sauce and tofu. Heat through gently, without boiling. Serve in small soup bowls.

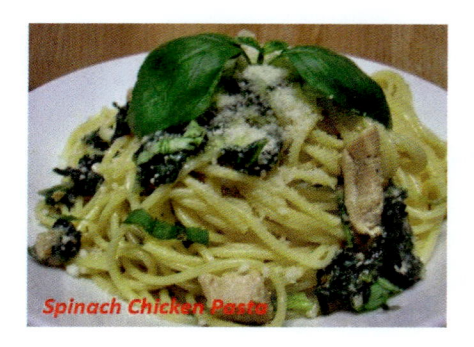

Spinach Chicken Pasta

Spinach Chicken Pasta

- 400g organic pasta, cooked
- 400g boneless skinless chicken breast, prepared and sliced
- 4 cloves garlic, minced
- 1 teaspoon red pepper flakes
- 2 lemons, juiced
- 1 cup parmesan, grated
- 1 cup spinach
- 3 tablespoons olive

Method

1. Heat garlic, oil, lemon juice, and red pepper over low heat for about 10 minutes. When a few minutes remain, add grated parmesan and stir as it melts.
2. Remove from heat and fold spinach into sauce until wilted.
   3. Toss pasta and chicken with sauce and top with lemon zest and parmesan.

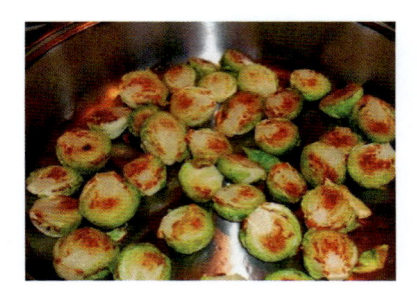

Apples and Brussels Sprouts

- 3 tablespoons butter
- 1/2 white onion, diced
- Salt, to taste
- 1 red apple, diced
- 450g brussel sprouts, bottoms trimmed, quartered
- 2 fresh sage leaves, thinly sliced
- 1/2 tsp fresh rosemary, chopped
- 2 tsp champagne vinegar
- 2 tsp honey

Method

1. Melt the butter in a large skillet over medium heat. Add the onion and a pinch of salt and cook until beginning to brown.
2. Add the apple and stir occasionally until the apple starts to brown.
3. Add the Brussels sprouts, pinch of salt, sage, rosemary and cook, stirring occasionally until sprouts are well browned. Careful not to overcook the Brussels sprouts taking away from their high nutrient content!
4. Add the champagne vinegar, honey. Adjust seasonings to taste..

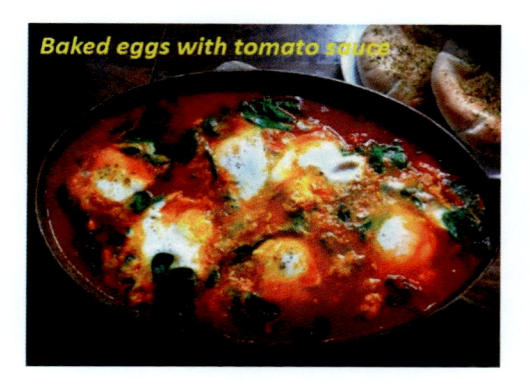

Baked eggs with tomato sauce

- 2 slices thick cut bacon cut into 1/4″ strips(optional)
- 1 shallot minced
- 2 Tbs parsley stems removed and chopped
- 5 ramps, bulbs minced, leaves chopped
- 1 1/2 C stewed tomatoes chopped
- salt and pepper to taste
- honey to taste (optional)
- 2-3 eggs
- ricotta insalata or other crumbly cheese

Method

1. Move your oven rack to the top position and turn on the broiler.
2. Add the bacon to a small oven safe pan and fry over medium heat until some oil renders out. Add the shallots and ramp bulbs and sauté until they are soft and fragrant. Add the parsley and ramp leaves and fry until they are just wilted. Add the tomatoes then salt and pepper to taste (you probably won't need much salt because stewed tomatoes usually have some salt

and the bacon and cheese will be salty). Taste the sauce, if it is too tart, add some honey until you're happy with it.

3. Use a spoon to make 2-3 wells in the tomato sauce with a spoon and drop an egg in each divet. Crumble some cheese on top and bring the sauce to a boil. When you see the bottoms of the eggs start to turn white, transfer the pan to the oven. Broil directly under the heating element for about a minute, or until the cheese is browned and the eggs have turned white on top.

4. Garnish your baked eggs with something green (parsley, basil, chives, scallions, or ramp leaves would all work) and serve on toasted bread. brown.

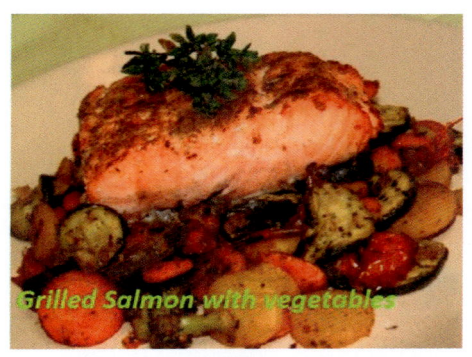

Grilled Salmon with vegetables

- 400g Pave de salmon
- 1 organic courgette
- 1 organic red pepper
- 1 red onion
- 1 carrot

For the accompanying sauce
- 1 yogurt
- 1 lemon
- parsley
- seasonings

Method

1. Make the lemon-parsley yogurt ahead by combining chopped parsley with the yogurt, adding fresh lemon juice and salt & pepper to taste.
2. Grill vegetables until you get nice grill marks. About 10 minutes depending on your grill.
3. Season the salmon with pepper and salt. Drizzle olive oil before adding to grill to prevent it from sticking.
4. Let grill until just done, middle of salmon is still pink.
5. Serve with yogurt dressing.

4 *LUTEAL PHASE*

Now is the time to load up on nutrients that encourage cell growth and keep hormones in check to prevent early miscarriage. The corpus luteum, which helps produce the progesterone necessary to sustain a pregnancy, is loaded with Beta-carotene, the powerful nutrient, which is commonly found in leafy greens as well as yellow and orange foods (carrots, cantaloupe and sweet potatoes).

One food that gets a lot of attention during this phase is pineapple. In addition to beta-carotene, pineapple contains a substance called bromelain, which has been shown to mildly support implantation through its anti-inflammatory properties.

This week is all about warming foods like soups and stews. The luteal phase is all about creating higher temperatures to help hold a pregnancy.

Avoid: Cold or raw foods, especially ice cream and frozen yogurt. The luteal phase is a time when you want to promote growth and expansion; cold constricts. Avoid or limit cow's milk and dairy.

As silly as it may sound remember to keep your body and particularly feet.

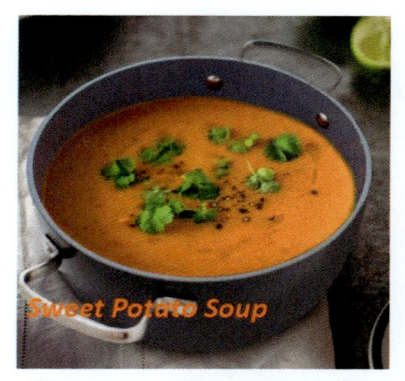

Sweet Potato Soup

- 3 large sweet potatoes, sliced and peeled
- 2 onions, finely sliced
- 4 large cloves of garlic
- 2 tsp ground coriander
- 2 tsp ground cumin
- 1 tsp paprika
- 1 tsp ground turmeric
- 1 tsp cayenne pepper
- 1 200ml tin coconut milk
- Juice of 1 lemon
- Salt, pepper and olive oil
- Fresh coriander to garnish

Method

1. Bake the peeled and sliced sweet potatoes, along with the whole garlic cloves in the oven for 30 minutes, sprinkle the chucks with oil, salt and pepper. Meanwhile, fry the onions, ground coriander, cumin, paprika, turmeric and cayenne pepper in a little olive oil. Once the sweet potato is cooked through blend it, together with the onions and garlic, until smooth.
2. Return the puree to the saucepan, add the coconut milk, lemon juice and a cup of water. Bring to the boil,

season to taste and serve with a little coriander to garnish.

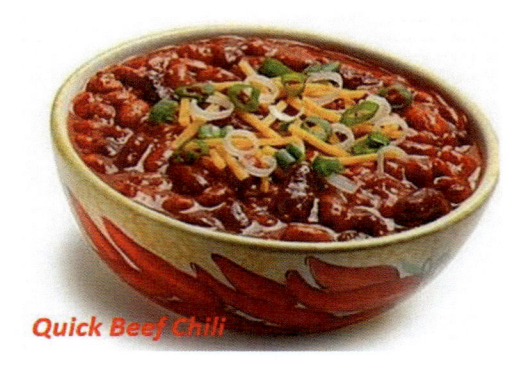

Quick Beef Chili

Quick Beef Chili

- 1 tablespoon vegetable oil
- 600g lean ground beef
- 1/2 cup chopped onion
- chili seasoning mix
- 1/2 cup water
- 1 tin organic diced tomatoes, undrained
- 1 can kidney beans or pinto beans, undrained
- 1 tablespoon brown sugar 2 tsp ground cumin
- 1 tsp paprika

Method

1. Spray skillet with nonstick cooking spray. Brown ground beef with onion. Add remaining ingredients. Cover and simmer for 20 minutes.

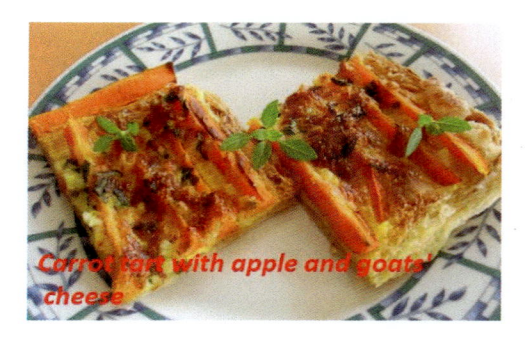

Carrot tart with apple and goats' cheese

Carrot tart with apple and goats' cheese

- 8 carrots
- 1 sheet puff pastry
- 1 onion halved and thinly sliced
- 1 cooking apple , peeled, cored, and sliced as thinly as possible
- 100 g goats cheese
- 100 g creme fraiche
- 150 ml carrot juice
- 3 eggs (be aware this dish serves 6 people)

Method

1. Boil the carrots in salted water for 8 minutes, until just tender. Drain and rinse under cold running water. Halve them lengthwise and set them aside.

2. Grease a 24cm tart pan with a removable bottom with a little butter. On a well-floured surface, roll out the puff pastry into a nice round slab the size of the pie

plate. Press the dough firmly into the plate and trim the edges neatly. With a fork, stab some holes in the bottom, then cover the dough and place the pie plate in the fridge for 30 minutes.

3. Preheat the oven to 180C/160C fan/gas 4. Arrange the onion and apple over the bottom of the pastry in the pie plate and place the halved carrots on top in a spoke pattern. Crumble the goats' cheese over the pie and in between the carrots.

4. In a medium bowl, whisk together the crème fraîche, carrot juice, eggs and season with salt and pepper. Pour the mixture over the carrots and sprinkle everything generously with pepper. Bake the pie on the lower rack of the oven for about 35 minutes, until golden brown.

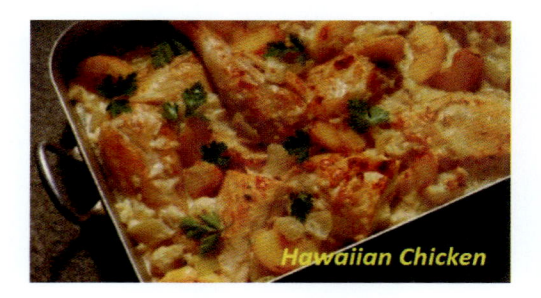

Hawaiian Chicken

- 5-6 boneless organic chicken breasts (approx 1200g)
- tin of pineapple slices, drained
- tin of mandarin oranges, drained
- 1/4 cup corn starch
- 1/2 cup brown sugar
- 1/2 cup soy sauce
- 1/4 cup lemon juice
- 1 tsp ground ginger
- salt/pepper, to taste preference (you can invite some friends for dinner, this dish will serve up to 6 people)

Method

1. Spray crock pot with non stick cooking spray or use liners. Place chicken in pot.
2. In a mixing bowl, whisk together corn starch, brown sugar, soy sauce, lemon juice, ginger and salt/pepper. Pour over chicken.
3. Next, pour in drained pineapple slices and mandarin oranges
4. Cover and cook on low for 4-5 hours.

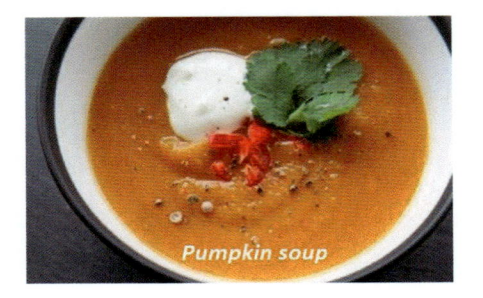

Pumpkin soup

- 1 red organic pumpkin (chopped in small block sized pieces)
- 1 onion (chopped very finely)
- 2 organic potatoes
- 1 tablespoon butter
- 1 pinch of salt
- 1 pinch of pepper
- cream (optional)

Method

1. Add butter in a saucepan and fry the chopped onions. Once onion turns a little translucent add the chopped potatoes and pumpkin. Let it cook for sometime on slow heat.
2. Then add water and bring the vegetables to a blow. Add salt and pepper to taste.
3. Once the vegetables are cooked let them cool. Grind them in a blender. Reheat in the same saucepan. Add some cream to taste. Serve with hot garlic bread.

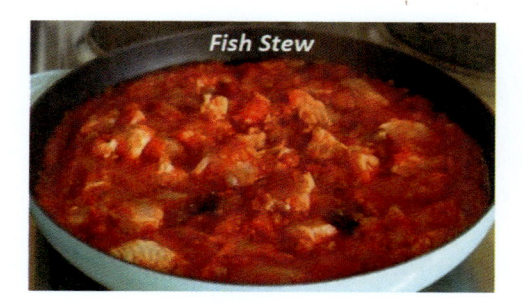

Fish Stew

- 6 Tbsp olive oil
- 1 cup of chopped onions
- 2 large garlic cloves, chopped
- 2/3 cup fresh parsley, chopped
- 1 cup of fresh chopped tomato (about 1 medium sized tomato)
- 2 teaspoons tomato paste
- 8 oz of clam juice (or shellfish stock)
- 1/2 cup dry white wine (like Sauvignon blanc)
- 1 1/2 lb fish fillets (use halibut, cod, sole, red snapper, sea bass), cut into 2-inch pieces
- Touch of dry oregano, Tabasco, thyme, pepper
- Salt

Method

1. Heat olive oil in large pot over medium-high heat. Add chopped onion and garlic and sauté 4 minutes. Add parsley and stir 2 minutes. Add tomato and tomato paste, and gently cook for 10 minutes.
2. Add clam juice, dry white wine, and fish and simmer until fish is cooked through, less than 10 minutes. Add seasoning. Salt to taste. Ladle into bowls and serve.

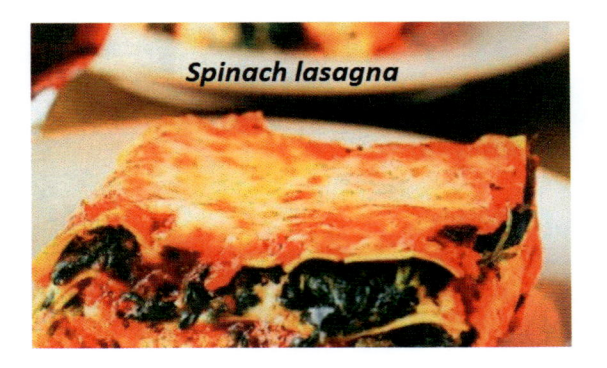

Spinach lasagna

- 750g Ricotta cheese or Fromage frais
- 125g Parmesan, freshly grated
- 1 large egg
- 1 liter chunky tomato pasta sauce
- 220g (12 sheets) no-precook egg lasagna
- 600g frozen chopped spinach, thawed and squeezed dry
- 250g mozzarella cheese, coarsely grated (serves 4-6)

Method

1. Preheat the oven to 180°C (gas 4). Mix together the ricotta, Parmesan and egg in a large bowl.
2. Spread 250ml of the pasta sauce over the base of a lightly oiled, large baking dish, measuring about 23 x 33cm and about 7cm deep.
3. Arrange three of the lasagna sheets side by side in the dish. Spread with a quarter of the ricotta mixture then top with a third of the spinach. Repeat layering twice

more with the sauce, lasagna, ricotta mixture and spinach. Top with remaining three sheets of lasagna.

4. Spread the remaining ricotta mixture and sauce over the top, then gently press the lasagna sheets down into the dish, so the sauce comes up around the sides. Cover the dish with foil.
5. Bake for 35 minutes, then uncover, sprinkle with the mozzarella and bake for a further 20 minutes until golden and bubbling.
6. Allow to stand for 10 minutes before cutting into rectangles to serve warm.

ABOUT THE AUTHOR

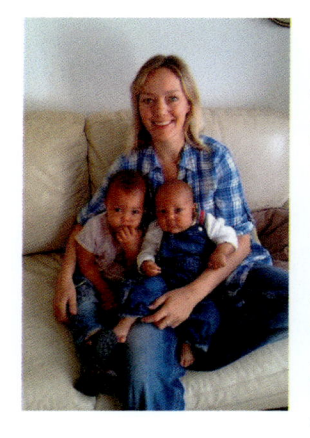

Pavla Kesslerova, author of 5 Simple Steps To Fertility was born 1973 in Czech Republic. After finishing A-levels in child care, child psychology and pedagogy she spent years traveling across Europe and America. In 2006 she settled in England. Until 2014 worked as a registered Domiciliary Care Manager in a company specialized in supporting young adults with Autism and Aspeger syndrome. She left her beloved job to stay at home with her two children.

Books:

5 SIMPLE STEPS TO FERTILITY: Pregnant naturally, after years of struggling with endometriosis (Baby at 40).

28 Day Fertility Diet

A-Z Pocket Guide For a First Time Dad

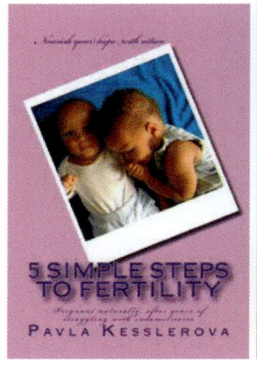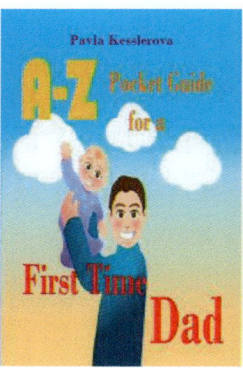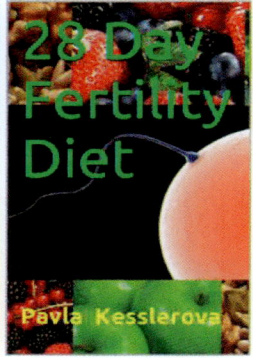

20289499R00028

Printed in Great Britain
by Amazon